NEUROFIBROMATOSIS MANAGEMENT DIET COOKBOOK

Nutrient Rich Recipes For Healthier

Living:

Boost Immunity And Manage

Symptoms Naturally:

Delicious Meals For Optimal Wellness

DR. SHAYLA LEWIS

Table of Contents

DISCLAIMER

Write a brief complete Disclaimer for my diet cook book telling them that the author is not in any association with any company, business or individual and also this book is written by the authors knowledge and understanding

The information provided in this diet cookbook is based on the author's personal knowledge and understanding. The author is not affiliated with, endorsed by, or associated with any company, business, or individual. The recipes and dietary advice contained within this book are intended for informational purposes only. Readers should consult with a healthcare professional or a registered dietitian before making any significant changes to their diet or lifestyle. The author assumes no responsibility for any adverse effects that may result from the use or misuse of the information contained in this book.

CHAPTER ONE

Understanding Neurofibromatosis: What You Should Know

Neurofibromatosis (NF) is a set of hereditary illnesses that result in the growth of tumors on nerve tissue. These tumors can result in a variety of health issues, including nerve damage, skin abnormalities, and visual impairments. It is critical to recognize indications and symptoms early on, such as café-au-lait spots, skin nodules, and bone deformities, to get appropriate medical attention and support.

Importance of Nutrition in Managing Neurofibromatosis

Nutrition is essential for managing neurofibromatosis since it promotes overall health and may alleviate symptoms. A well-balanced diet high in fruits, vegetables, lean proteins, and whole grains can offer critical nutrients while limiting consumption of processed foods and carbohydrates. Furthermore, certain dietary changes, such as limiting coffee and alcohol consumption, may help manage symptoms such as pain and inflammation.

Addressing Misconceptions About Dietary Restrictions

There are several misconceptions about dietary limitations for people with neurofibromatosis. While there is no special "NF diet," it is critical to prioritize general good eating habits over rigid restrictions. Contrary to popular perception, there is no substantial evidence that specific foods cause the development or aggravation of neurofibromatosis symptoms. Instead, eating a balanced diet suited to individual needs can improve general health.

This cookbook is a useful resource for those living with neurofibromatosis, providing nutritious and delicious dishes adapted to their specific dietary needs and tastes.

From simple breakfast options to fulfilling main dishes and snacks, each recipe is intended to deliver critical nutrients while accommodating a variety of taste preferences and dietary limitations. By including these dishes in your meal plan, you may help your journey to better health and well-being.

Nutritional Influence on Neurofibromatosis

Understanding how diet affects your neurofibromatosis is critical for managing it. By investigating the link between your food and nerve pain, you may begin making informed decisions that benefit your health. Furthermore, understanding the role of inflammation and how specific foods might worsen or alleviate it can have a big impact on your overall health. Incorporating antioxidant-rich foods into your diet will help with healing and reducing oxidative stress on your body, whilst eating low-carb meals helps stabilize blood sugar levels, which is critical for managing neurofibromatosis symptoms. Tailoring your diet to your specific needs and symptoms can significantly enhance your overall health and quality of life.

Investigating the relationship between nutrition and nerve pain.

Understanding how your diet impacts nerve pain is crucial for managing neurofibromatosis. Certain foods can increase or alleviate nerve pain, so it's critical to identify and eliminate irritants from your diet. Keeping a food diary and tracking how different foods affect your symptoms allows you to make informed decisions to reduce discomfort and enhance your quality of life. Experimenting with different dietary techniques, such as decreasing inflammatory foods and including nerve-friendly nutrients, can help you figure out what works best for controlling your neurofibromatosis symptoms.

Understanding inflammation and its impact on the body.

Inflammation is a major factor in neurofibromatosis, and understanding how it affects your body is critical for controlling the condition. Certain meals might cause inflammation, which worsens symptoms like pain and discomfort. Adopting an anti-inflammatory diet rich in fruits, vegetables, and omega-3 fatty acids can help reduce inflammation and relieve neurofibromatosis symptoms. Furthermore, lifestyle variables such as stress management and regular exercise can help to reduce inflammation and improve overall health.

Antioxidants are important in supporting recovery.

Consuming antioxidants is essential for boosting healing and treating neurofibromatosis symptoms. Antioxidants aid in battling oxidative stress created by free radicals, which can damage cells and increase the condition's symptoms. Consuming a diet rich in colorful fruits and vegetables, as well as foods high in vitamins C and E, will enhance your antioxidant intake and assist your body's natural healing processes. Incorporating antioxidant-rich herbs and spices like turmeric and ginger can also help your body mend and recover from neurofibromatosis symptoms.

CHAPTER TWO

How low-carb diets can help regulate blood sugar levels

Stabilizing blood sugar levels is critical for controlling neurofibromatosis symptoms, and following a low-carb diet can help with this. Carbohydrates are known to produce blood sugar increases, which can worsen symptoms like weariness and weakness. By limiting your intake of refined carbohydrates and replacing them with complex carbs and high-fiber foods, you can help prevent blood sugar fluctuations and maintain steady energy levels all day. Incorporating lean proteins and healthy fats into your meals can also help decrease carbohydrate absorption, which can help regulate blood sugar and manage symptoms.

Getting Started: Essential Kitchen Tools and Ingredients

Equip your kitchen with the necessary instruments for efficient cooking. Invest in the basics, such as a high-quality chef's knife, cutting board, and pots and pans. Stock your pantry with healthful essentials such as whole grains, legumes, nuts, and seeds. Learn how to decipher ingredient labels so you may make more informed food decisions. When grocery shopping, prioritize cost-effective options without sacrificing quality. Create a meal plan based on your dietary needs and tastes for a successful culinary trip.

Understanding peripheral neuropathy

Learn the fundamentals of peripheral neuropathy, a disorder that affects nerves outside the brain and spinal cord. Learn about its causes, symptoms, and potential problems to help you manage the illness. Investigate treatment alternatives, including medication, physical therapy, and lifestyle changes, to relieve pain and enhance quality of life.

Neurofibromatosis Management Diet

Learn about the specifics of managing neurofibromatosis through food. Discover how nutrition can help alleviate symptoms and improve overall health. Investigate dietary measures such as adding anti-inflammatory foods, eating a balanced diet high in fruits, vegetables, lean meats, and healthy fats, and minimizing processed foods and sugar consumption. Learn how to prepare delicious and nutritious meals that promote health while accommodating dietary constraints.

Cookbook Creation

Begin the process of constructing a neurofibromatosis treatment diet cookbook that is suited to your specific needs. Compile a collection of recipes that correspond to your food choices and health goals. Experiment with different flavors, textures, and cooking methods to keep meals interesting and pleasant. Consider integrating meal preparation suggestions, nutritional information, and personal anecdotes to increase the cookbook's value and appeal.

Putting It All Together

Incorporate the knowledge obtained into your regular habits. Implement techniques for controlling peripheral neuropathy symptoms, such as nutrition, lifestyle changes, and medical therapies. Use the cookbook to plan and create nutritious meals that promote overall health and wellness. Stay committed to the trip, making modifications as needed and enjoying accomplishments along the way.

Introduction to Basic Cooking Methods: Begin by learning the fundamentals of cooking methods such as sautéing, baking, and grilling. Sauteing cooks food fast in a tiny amount of oil over high heat, whereas baking cooks food in an oven using dry heat. Grilling, on the other hand, is the process of cooking food over direct heat, typically using a grill or barbecue. Understanding these techniques creates the groundwork for preparing delicious and nutritious meals.

Mastering meal planning and batch cooking will simplify your culinary routine. Spend some time planning your weekly meals and preparing materials ahead of time to save time on hectic weekdays. Batch cooking entails preparing huge amounts of food at once and portioning it for future meals. This method not only saves time but also guarantees that you have nutritious options on hand when hunger strikes.

Portion Control and Serving Sizes: Understanding portion control is essential for keeping a balanced diet. Understand the recommended serving sizes for each food group and use measuring instruments such as cups and scales to avoid overeating. It's also useful to visualize portion sizes with common things like a deck of cards or your fist. Mastering portion management allows you to better regulate your calorie intake and maintain a healthy weight.

Incorporating Flavour Without Unhealthy Additions: By incorporating natural flavors and herbs, you may improve the taste of your foods without using harmful additives. Use fresh herbs like basil, parsley, and cilantro to add depth and richness to your dishes. Spices such as paprika, cumin, and turmeric can help you produce robust and vibrant flavors without using too much salt or sugar. By experimenting with different flavor combinations, you may make your cooking more pleasant and healthier.

Cooking should be enjoyable and stress-free. Before you begin cooking, organize your kitchen and gather all of the necessary supplies and tools to create a calm atmosphere. To generate a happy mood, play your favorite music or podcast, and make cooking a social activity by involving family members or friends. Don't be scared to explore and make errors; cooking is about learning and having fun along the way.

Quick and easy breakfast options for busy mornings: We realize how stressful mornings can be, so we've chosen a list of breakfast options that are both nutritious and quick to make. Consider overnight oats that you can make the night before, grab-and-go fruit and nut bars, or even pre-made smoothie packs that you can blend in minutes. These breakfast options do not require much cooking or preparation, making them ideal for hectic mornings when every minute matters.

Balancing protein, healthy fats, and fiber for sustained energy: An important component of a nutritious breakfast is ensuring that it delivers long-lasting energy to get you through the morning. We emphasize the necessity of balancing macronutrients such as protein, healthy fats, and fiber to do this. Incorporating protein sources such as eggs, Greek yogurt, or plant-based protein powders helps you stay full and happy. Healthy fats like nuts, seeds, and avocados give a consistent source of energy, but fiber-rich meals like whole grains, fruits, and vegetables improve digestion and promote satiety.

Smoothies are a great breakfast option since they include a variety of nutrients in one handy drink. This section contains a variety of smoothie recipes tailored to different tastes and nutritional preferences. There's something for everyone, from classic green smoothies full of healthy greens and strawberries to decadent chocolate peanut butter masterpieces. These meals not only taste delicious, but they also deliver a healthy dose of vitamins, minerals, and antioxidants.

Creative muesli and grain bowl ideas: Muesli and grain bowls are versatile breakfast options that may be tailored to your tastes and nutritional requirements. We have a variety of unique solutions to improve your morning muesli or grain bowl game. Consider topping your oats with fresh fruit, almonds, and honey for a pleasant and nutritious start to the day. Alternatively, try savory grain bowls with roasted veggies, a poached egg, and a sprinkle of cheese for a hearty and fulfilling breakfast alternative. With these inventive ideas, you'll never get bored with your morning oats or grains.

CHAPTER THREE

 Finally, we understand that prioritizing breakfast in your routine might be difficult at times, especially if you have a hectic schedule. That is why we offer practical advice to help you schedule time for breakfast and start your day off right. Whether it's prepping items ahead of time, scheduling dedicated breakfast time, or encouraging family members to share breakfast tasks, we have methods to make breakfast a seamless and joyful part of your daily routine. By following these suggestions, you'll find it easier than ever to prioritize breakfast and gain the benefits of beginning your day with a nutritious meal.

Salad recipes that are both simple and satisfying: Use a range of fresh ingredients, such as leafy greens, lean proteins like grilled chicken or tofu, and colorful veggies like tomatoes, cucumbers, and bell peppers. Dress them with homemade vinaigrettes or light dressings for more flavor without the calories.

Flavorful sandwich and wrap ideas: Make sandwiches or wraps with whole grain bread or wraps as the base. Fill them with lean protein sources like turkey or tuna, as well as plenty of greens like lettuce, spinach, and avocado. Instead of high-calorie spreads or sauces, try mustard, hummus, or salsa to add flavor.

one-pot dishes with minimum cleanup. Consider soups, stews, or stir-fries, which may be filled with vegetables, protein, and whole grains to make a complete meal in one pot.

Incorporating leftovers into excellent lunch options: Don't waste leftovers; instead, repurpose them into inventive and appetizing lunch dishes. For a quick and easy meal, toss leftover grilled chicken or roasted vegetables into salads, wraps, or grain bowls.

Strategies for staying energized throughout the day: To sustain energy levels, eat balanced meals with a variety of proteins, healthy fats, and complex carbohydrates. Snack on nutrient-dense foods such as nuts, fruits, or yogurt in between meals to stave off hunger and maintain energy levels until the next meal.

Wholesome Dinners: Finishing the Day on a High Note

Making healthful dinners is essential for general well-being. This section includes a variety of nutrient-dense recipes designed to improve health. You may make nutrient-dense meals by combining various proteins, vegetables, and grains. From colorful stir-fries to hearty skillet meals, these dishes guarantee both flavor and nutrition. Furthermore, by embracing healthy comfort food makeovers, you may savor familiar flavors without guilt. Combining these meals with mindful eating habits creates a peaceful dining experience, encouraging relaxation after a long day.

Nutrient-dense meal recipes for maximum wellness.

Unlocking the potential of nutrient-dense meal recipes is critical to achieving peak health. This section features a selection of meticulously picked recipes designed to maximize nutritional benefits. These recipes provide necessary vitamins and minerals by combining a variety of proteins, veggies, and grains. From flavorful salads to healthful grain bowls, each recipe exemplifies nourishment and well-being. Including these nutrient-dense meals in your diet allows you to prioritize health without sacrificing taste.

Including a range of proteins, veggies, and grains.

Diversifying your dinner plate with a variety of proteins, veggies, and grains creates the groundwork for a balanced and nutritious diet. This part emphasizes the need to include a range of various food groups to improve nutrition. You may prepare satisfying and healthy meals by incorporating proteins such as lean meats, lentils, and tofu, as well as a colorful array of vegetables and beneficial grains such as quinoa and brown rice. This technique not only provides a well-rounded diet but also adds a variety of flavors and textures to satisfy the palette.

Delicious stir-fries and skillet dinners.

Enhance your supper repertoire with the ease and vibrancy of tasty stir-fry and skillet dishes. This area presents a variety of dishes that claim to tantalize your taste senses while making meal preparation easier. These dishes are flavorful and nutritious since they make use of fresh ingredients and aromatic spices. Whether you like a sizzling stir-fry loaded with crisp vegetables and delicate protein, or a hearty skillet supper bursting with healthful grains and savory sauces, these dishes provide a quick and delicious option for hectic evenings.

CHAPTER FOUR
Healthy Comfort Food Makeovers

With these inventive comfort food makeovers, you may enjoy the comfortable embrace of classic flavors while also prioritizing your health. This series reimagines classic recipes from the viewpoint of nutrition and well-being, demonstrating that healthy eating can still be genuinely pleasurable.

From guilt-free versions of creamy pasta dishes to healthy variations of classic casseroles, these recipes combine nostalgia with nourishment. You may enjoy the warmth and satisfaction of comfort food without sacrificing your health objectives by making thoughtful ingredient changes and combining nutrient-rich ingredients.

Find nutritious snack options to fulfill desires without disrupting your neurofibromatosis management diet. Instead of going for packaged snacks, try nutrient-dense alternatives such as apple slices with almond butter, Greek yogurt with berries, or a handful of mixed nuts. These snacks have a balanced amount of protein, healthy fats, and carbohydrates, keeping you satiated and energized between meals while also supporting your health goals.

Prepare delicious dips and spreads for entertaining without compromising your diet. Make simple and tasty dips and spreads like hummus, guacamole, or tzatziki with fresh ingredients. Pair them with crisp vegetable sticks or whole grain crackers for a filling snack that everyone will like. These handmade selections are lower in salt and include no additives, making them a healthier choice for entertaining.

For guilt-free snacking, try homemade chips and vegetarian crisps. Avoid store-bought chips that are high in unhealthy fats and preservatives and instead make your own at home. Slice sweet potatoes, beets, or kale thinly, mix with olive oil and spices, and bake until crispy. These homemade chips and veggie crisps are high in vitamins and minerals, low in calories, and include no artificial chemicals, making them a guilt-free snack alternative.

Enhance your meals with nutritious side dishes that assist your neurofibromatosis management objectives. Fill your plate with colorful veggies, such as roasted broccoli, sautéed spinach, or grilled asparagus, to boost your fiber, vitamin, and antioxidant intake. Incorporate complete grains such as quinoa, brown rice, or farro to increase protein and complex carbohydrate content. These nutritious sides not only add flavor and diversity to your meals, but they also help you feel better overall.

Manage neurofibromatosis through mindful snacking and portion control strategies. Pay attention to your hunger cues and choose snacks that nourish your body without overeating.

To avoid mindless snacking, portion snacks into tiny dishes or containers. Also, avoid eating directly from the packet. Incorporate protein and fiber into your snacks to help you feel fuller for longer and avoid overeating. Adopting these tactics allows you to have enjoyable snacks while adhering to your neurofibromatosis management diet.

Indulge in sweet treats without guilt.

Looking for a sweet treat? Discover a world of guilt-free enjoyment with healthier dessert alternatives. There are numerous ways to enjoy sweets without compromising your health goals, including replacing refined sugars with natural alternatives such as honey or maple syrup, as well as incorporating whole grains and fruits.

Experiment with baking suggestions like lowering sugar and fat content by using applesauce or mashed bananas. Get inventive with fruit-based desserts, such as grilled peaches drizzled with balsamic sauce or a crisp fruit salad with a dash of mint. And don't worry, chocolate lovers: indulge in decadent yet nutritious chocolate recipes that will satisfy your desires while also giving antioxidants and joy. With these simple changes and recipes, indulging your sugar desire has never been more guilt-free!

Satisfying sweet desires doesn't have to compromise your health goals. Explore a variety of healthy dessert options that will satisfy your taste senses while also making your body feel good. Replace processed sugars with natural sweeteners such as honey, maple syrup, or dates to offer sweetness without guilt.

To increase nutrient intake, try whole grains and alternative flours such as almond or coconut flour. To keep you feeling fuller for longer, choose fiber and protein-rich treats like chia seed pudding or Greek yogurt with fresh fruit and a sprinkle of honey. You can satisfy your appetites without jeopardizing your healthy eating habits by making minor adjustments to your dessert choices.

Tips for baking with less sugar and fat.

Do you enjoy baking but wish to reduce sugar and fat? Discover easy yet effective baking strategies for reducing the sugar and fat content of your favorite foods without sacrificing flavor. Begin by reducing the amount of sugar in your recipes by a third, then gradually decrease it as your taste buds adjust.

Replace butter or oil with healthy alternatives such as applesauce, mashed bananas, or Greek yogurt to add moisture without the added fat. Experiment with natural flavor enhancers such as vanilla essence, cinnamon, or nutmeg to boost the flavor without using sugar. By adding these baking methods into your routine, you may indulge in your favorite baked items guilt-free.

Innovative fruit-based treats for a pleasant taste.

Looking for a tasty and nutritious treat? Explore the world of innovative fruit-based sweets that will fulfill your sweet desire without guilt.

 From basic fruit salads to more sophisticated creations such as grilled fruit skewers or fruit parfaits, there are limitless things to try. Experiment with different fruit combinations to make colorful and savory sweets that are as visually appealing as they are tasty. Experiment with unusual fruits like mangoes, kiwis, and papayas, or stick to traditional favorites like strawberries, blueberries, and bananas. Whether you're looking for a light dessert after dinner or a sweet snack, fruit-based delights are sure to satisfy.

Can chocolate be both delicious and nutritious? Indulge your chocolate cravings with recipes that are both tasty and nutritious. Explore the world of dark chocolate, which has more antioxidants and less sugar than milk chocolate.

Make a batch of handmade chocolate bark with nuts and dried fruit for a deliciously crispy dessert. Dive into a bowl of chocolate avocado mousse for a creamy and delicious dessert full of healthy fats. Alternatively, satiate your sweet taste with a guilt-free chocolate smoothie made from cocoa powder, banana, and almond milk. These luscious yet nutritious chocolate dishes allow you to indulge without feeling guilty.

Grilled salmon with lemon and dill: High in omega-3 anti-inflammatory fatty acids.

Quinoa Salad with Roasted Veggies: Quinoa contains protein and fiber, while roasted veggies supply vitamins and minerals.

Turmeric Chicken Stir-Fry: Turmeric includes curcumin, which has anti-inflammatory properties.

Lentils are high in protein and fiber, and vegetables contain important minerals.

Baked Sweet Potato with Black Beans and Avocado: Sweet potatoes are high in antioxidants, and black beans provide protein and fiber.

Spinach & Mushroom Omelette: Eggs are abundant in protein and nutrients, while the spinach and mushrooms add vitamins and minerals.

Grilled Chicken Caesar Salad: Grilled chicken is a lean protein source, and the salad includes a variety of veggies and a light dressing.

Sautéed Shrimp with Garlic and Broccoli: Shrimp is low in fat and calories but high in protein when combined with nutrient-dense broccoli.

Mediterranean Chickpea Salad: Chickpeas are high in protein and fiber, so combine them with fresh veggies and a mild vinaigrette.

Baked Cod with Tomatoes and Basil: Cod is a lean protein source, while tomatoes and basil add antioxidants and flavor.

Here's a 30-day meal plan that includes these meals.

Week 1:

Day 1: Grilled salmon with lemon and dill, quinoa salad.

Day 2: Turmeric Chicken Stir-Fry.

Day 3: Vegetable Lentil Soup with Whole Grain Bread.

Day 4: Baked sweet potatoes with black beans and avocado.

Day 5: Spinach and Mushroom Omelette with Whole Grain Toast.

Day 6: Grilled chicken Caesar salad.

Day 7: Sautéed Shrimp with Garlic and Broccoli, Brown Rice.

Week 2:

Repeat Week 1, modifying portions and sides as needed.

Week 3:

Day 15: Mediterranean Chickpea Salad.

Day 16: Baked cod with tomato and basil, steamed green beans.

Day 17: Grilled salmon with lemon and dill, quinoa salad.

Day 18: Turmeric Chicken Stir-Fry.

Day 19: Vegetable Lentil Soup with Whole Grain Bread.

Day 20: Baked sweet potatoes with black beans and avocado.

Day 21: Spinach and Mushroom Omelette with Whole Grain Toast.

Week 4:

Repeat Week 3, changing portions and sides accordingly.

Remember to eat snacks like fresh fruits, almonds, or yogurt in between meals to stay energized and deliver extra nutrients. Consult a healthcare practitioner or certified dietitian for personalized dietary recommendations based on your specific health needs and preferences.

Finally, the "Neurofibromatosis Management Diet Cookbook" provides a thorough guide for those navigating the intricacies of managing Neurofibromatosis (NF) with dietary interventions. Neurofibromatosis, a hereditary illness affecting the nervous system, necessitates a multidisciplinary approach to therapy, and nutrition is critical in maintaining general health and well-being.

This cookbook emphasizes the necessity of including nutrient-dense foods with anti-inflammatory and antioxidant characteristics, which can help alleviate symptoms associated with NF. Each recipe has been carefully chosen to supply critical nutrients while also providing delicious and filling meal options.

Recipes throughout the cookbook include omega-3 fatty acid-rich items like salmon and walnuts, which have been demonstrated to have anti-inflammatory properties that may assist people with NF. Furthermore, the incorporation of colorful fruits and vegetables guarantees a varied range of vitamins, minerals, and phytonutrients required for good health.

Individuals with Neurofibromatosis can achieve a balanced and satisfying diet that meets their specific nutritional requirements by following the meal plans suggested in this cookbook. The recipes range from nourishing soups to vivid salads and tasty protein dishes, providing variety and adaptability to suit varied tastes and preferences.

Furthermore, this cookbook is a helpful resource for not only people with NF but also their carers and healthcare practitioners. It offers practical advice on meal planning, grocery shopping, and food preparation procedures that are adapted to the unique nutritional needs of people with NF.

Overall, the "Neurofibromatosis Management Diet Cookbook" provides patients with the knowledge and tools they need to make informed dietary decisions that will improve their health and quality of life. Individuals with Neurofibromatosis can take proactive actions to manage their illness and improve

their well-being by eating a balanced and
tasty diet.

THE END

www.ingramcontent.com/pod-product-compliance
Lightning Source LLC
Chambersburg PA
CBHW061313250726
48653CB00002B/926